99 Tips
to Reset the Table

Parenting in a Society Obsessed with
Food, Weight, Obesity, & Body Image

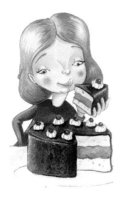

by Iréné Celcer

illustrated by
Horacio Gatto

Graphite

PUBLISHED BY GRAPHITE PRESS

Copyright © 2014 by Iréné Celcer
Illustrations Copyright © 2014 by Graphite Press

www.graphitepress.com

The contents of this publication are for informational purposes only, and not a substitute for professional medical or mental health advice. The author and publisher disclaim any liability with regard to the use of such contents. Readers should consult appropriate professionals on any matter relating to their health and well-being.

LIBRARY OF CONGRESS CATALOGING-IN-PUBLICATION DATA

Celcer, Iréné.
99 tips to reset the table : parenting in a society obsessed with food, weight, obesity, & body image
/ by Iréné Celcer ; illustrated by Horacio Gatto.
pages cm
Summary: "Parenting advice for a lifestyle that promotes healthy eating, encourages a positive body image, and supports the psychological well-being of children and family"—Provided by publisher.
ISBN 978-1-938313-01-1 (pbk. : alk. paper) —
ISBN 978-1-938313-02-8 (Spanish Language)
1. Parenting. 2. Children—Nutrition. 3. Body image.
I. Title. II. Title: Ninety nine tips to reset the table.
HQ755.8.C4295 2014
649'.1—dc23
2013017157

FIRST EDITION

To Tadeo Celcer,
who taught me the joy of chocolate,
and almost everything I know.

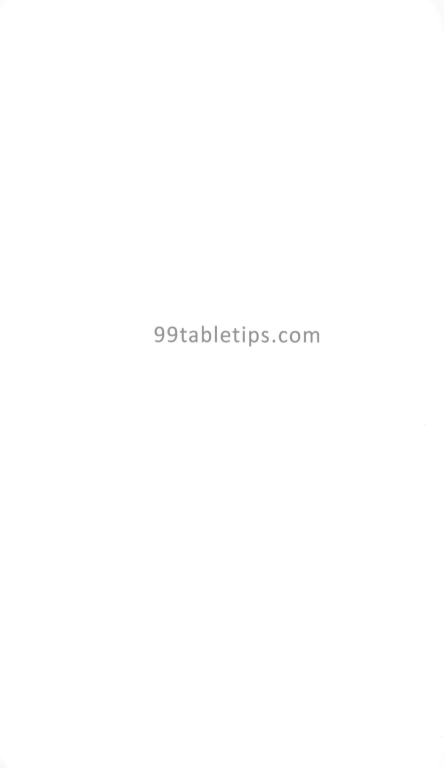
99tabletips.com

Contents

About this Book

This book is about learning how to develop a family lifestyle that promotes healthy and nutritious eating, encourages a positive body image, and supports parental responses that are beneficial to the psychological well-being of your children. Like the injections the pediatrician gave your children when they were babies, these tips will help inoculate your children against future problems with eating, food and body image.

Achieving a healthy family lifestyle begins with good parenting. However, good parenting in these areas is not necessarily instinctual. Many times, we must unlearn what was taught to us as children and learn new approaches that make us better parents.

"I am already a good parent who knows about healthy foods," you say? Well, of course you are! But even if we're good at parenting, we can always enhance our existing knowledge with strategies and techniques that serve to sharpen our skills. By wanting to learn more about this topic, I applaud your efforts!

The Illustrations & Language

The illustrations in this book evolved from the combined imaginations of the illustrator and author. The author's clinical experience guided how eating problems were configured and presented through language. And the illustrator interpreted the author's intent in ways that brought the content to life.

Because this book intends to bring joy to the experience of eating in a family, we included illustrations that are colorful, semi-realistic, caricatural, or cartoon-like in style. Their variety is designed to respectfully depict all kinds of families, as well as people from varying socioeconomic backgrounds, races, and cultures. We did not intend for the illustrations to show any particular cultural ideal with respect to body shape or size. Although some images illustrate clinical problems, our intention was to portray all kinds of bodies, representing our full respect for the diversity of the human condition.

We have been mindful to balance genders, problems and disorders, but perfect equality is impossible. Moreover, eating problems and disorders, food issues, and home cooking are imbalanced phenomena, with women bearing the preponderance of experience. We apologize to the reader who might find words, phrases or illustrations politically incorrect or potentially offensive, and we assure them that we have tried our best to be sensitive and fair.

Acknowledgments

The list of people who have inspired this book is longer than the list of tips themselves, so I could not possibly list them all. However, my gratitude is immeasurable, for they have brought the brightest insight and deepest warmth to this endeavor.

I am indebted to all my patients, whose stories about food and eating have helped me understand the unique needs of children, tweens and teens. Through the tips in this book, I have tried to convey what parents can offer to the family experience so that the practice of eating is a happy and healthy one. All my patients' voices remain in my heart, and I feel privileged and honored that they have let me into their lives. Although I cannot mention you by name, you know who you are—my deepest thanks!

To my dear friend Mimo Tolchinsky, my thanks run deep. We have been friends forever and it will remain this way forever forward. Our many conversations and her invaluable input and ideas on issues surrounding children and food have infused this book with wisdom and humor. She is one of those people whose knowledge about children seems infinite!

My unending thanks go to Kathleen Barkley, whose keen understanding of eating problems and parenting issues have delighted me during our morning walks. She has been a staunch supporter of this book and its ideas since I

first thought of writing it. I can't thank her enough for her
optimism and enthusiasm.

In the literary sphere, I wish to thank the editors at
Graphite Press for their trust and steadfast support of
my writing projects. I consider Graphite Press my writing
home.

In the media sphere, Cristina Varela and Luis Enrique
Angió have provided me with a special outlet on their radio
show, Oid Mortales, in spite of the miles that separate us,
and the times that constrain us. It is on their show that
we first broadcast some of the early ideas I developed for
this book, and where my certainty for the need of a Spanish language translation solidified. How can I thank them
enough?

In the clinical sphere, there are two central concepts
that are blended into this book of tips. The first is that one
should eat in response to physical hunger. And the second
is that diets do not work. The original ideas behind these
concepts were not mine. They were taught to me more
than two decades ago when I attended a group at The
Women's Therapy Centre to address my own eating. To the
pioneers who created the Centre in London and New York
City—Carol Bloom, Susie Orbach, and Luise Eichenbaum—I
feel incredibly indebted. I will never forget Susan Gutwill
whose teaching felt like magic! Jane R. Hirschmann and
Lela Zaphiropoulos also teach this approach in their book
Are You Hungry? (Random House, 1985), which has become an inspiration to many who work with children and
families. But, I owe my greatest gratitude to Carol Bloom,
who guided me with unparalleled support and assistance;
it is because of her that I am able to write for you today.

Some of those who helped me set the table for this
book are also those who help me set the table at home—
my beloved family. Of course what better acknowledgment
could there be, given that this book is all about family!

While writing different tips and chapters, my sister

and I had the deepest and most amazing conversations on body image, self, and psychoanalytic theory. She never ceases to amaze me with her wit and brilliance. Our sisterhood is a gift!

My nieces Alejandra, Florencia and Lucía Bonells have graciously offered their thoughts that led to the Spanish language title for this book. Alejandra shared her truly invaluable knowledge about food and the art of eating through her wonderful tweets and re-tweets; Flor brought her knowledge of the world of nutrition and dieting to the table, which was equally priceless. And Lucía's lucid use of language and grammar was invaluable; she has so much cultural awareness for a young woman and I love her for sharing it with me.

Ezequiel Boaglio has been the one person who has hit the jackpot for the title of this book. His accurate observations, thoughtful remarks and intelligent comments made me appreciate him in a whole new light. I thought he was a computer whiz. Now I know he is also a proficient authority on language, not to mention kind and generous with his time. Ezequiel, I am impressed!

To my father, although not involved in my everyday writing, was always present by example, braveness, and his three C's: *Constancia*, *Criterio*, and *Coraje*. Without constancy, good judgment and courage, I would not have been able to make it through the many obstacles and delays involved in publishing this book. It was through his daily example of perseverance that I have been able to bring this book to completion. I thank him sincerely, and love him deeply.

At last I come to my husband and my daughter. How can I describe my thanks to them? My daughter is smart and kind and lovely—all I could ever have hoped for in a daughter. She bravely lets me know when what I say is not in sync with what I do. And, of course, she has been right every time! With a smile I say, "Sophie, always stand up for what you believe in, just as you stood up for every Oreo and chocolate-anything you claimed as yours along the way. You go girl!"

My heartfelt thanks extend to my husband, who has been amazingly helpful during the writing of this book, with everything I needed from finding articles and references to washing dishes. Although we have not always seen eye to eye on the "food thing," I appreciate that he is secure enough to let me know, trusted me enough to defer, and loves me enough to let it be. And although he loves gourmet food, never once has he objected to leftovers or pizza. From day one I knew that I was lucky to have him at my table! Thanks—I love you!

Setting the Table

Given the significant challenges posed by eating disorders and obesity in our society, and given the often conflicting and confusing information available on how to prevent and combat them, it became unmistakably clear to me that children, parents, and families could benefit from guidance on these topics. Parents of young children, tweens and teens seemed hungry for a way to navigate the pressures of our culture concerning food, eating, and body image.

I see it all over the place—at home, at school, at work, on play dates, and in many other social situations with family, friends, or acquaintances. Everyone is bombarded with pressures to eat (or not eat) in ways that have nothing to do with simple hunger.

Parents are at a loss about what to do. They sometimes feel trapped in an impossible bind: Kids need to eat, but how do you go about feeding them nutritious food in a healthy manner without moving to a deserted island? News reports about the perils of obesity in children, coupled with worries about eating disorders and uncertainties about how to avoid body image problems and low self-esteem, seem omnipresent. More than a fair share of such issues are uncovered daily in the celebrities our daughters and sons admire as they follow stories on television, in the movies, and in social media.

Around every corner there lurks some kind of allur-
ing but risky food situation. You'll find a fast food joint
that promises delicious and inexpensive food, which also
happens to be a social gathering spot for your tweens or
teens. In a magazine you'll read about a new, chemically
engineered food that is scrumptiously delicious. And on
the same page you'll find new size 2 jeans that your daughter covets, worn by a size 2 model with perfect skin.

Although the words "diet" and "dieting" are démodé
these days, the concept is still alive and well. Strategies for
eating via specific meal plans are often advertised by com-
panies that make their money at the expense of people
feeling bad about their physiques. Although such compa-
nies no longer talk about "diets," they hide their money-
making goals behind claims of improved health and fitness.
So the pressure to diet still exists today, although it may no
longer go by that name.

Women, men, and even children are coerced by media, social, and cultural forces to adjust their eating in a
manner that's inconsistent with their own biology. You feel
compelled to be healthy, strong, thin, cool, a good athlete,
good looking at 20, 30, 40, or 50, or driven to dance some
other twist designed to appeal to your personal or social
insecurities. Instead of eating because it's instinctive—according to a built-in desire designed by nature—we eat to
achieve goals that have nothing to do with eating at all!

Mass quantities of fatty foods are everywhere you turn,
coupled with huge advertisements on the value of a "slim"
and "healthy" body. How do you deal with this paradox if
you are a child, a tween or a teen? And if you are a parent,
how do you reconcile these contradictions without moving
to an all-organic farm? Add to this the need for a full-time,
live-in dermatologist for the pimples, and you get my drift.
These are the kind of challenges that prompted me to
write this book—to help families reclaim the joy of eating
so that such struggles do not become a part their daily

domestic menu.

Why Tips?

When I began thinking about this book, I wondered how you, the parents, would ever find the time to read a book about eating when you barely have time to breathe, let alone eat! Parents are busy working, cooking, transporting children around town, attending school activities, picking up laundry, fixing the car, trying to manage their family's emotional life—not to mention cooking. Believe me—as a parent, I know! And if you are a single parent, things are exponentially busier and more complicated.

So writing a book of succinct tips that you could easily digest, instead of one with lengthy chapters that would take forever to read, seemed like a good idea. Many of the tips you'll find in this book come from questions that parents have posed to me over my many years of practice. Is it ever possible to feed our children good quality meals when our grocery stores are inundated with rows and rows of processed foods? Is it okay to eat dessert every day? How do we respond to demands for gum, ice cream, or potato chips? What do we say when our son begs, "But Justin's parents let him"? How do we navigate our own eating issues as parents, while ensuring a healthy pathway for our daughters?

Answers to these questions will help you *enhance* the pleasure and normality of family life—to add a sparkle of fun and happiness to the mundane activity of eating. I'd like these tips to add an element of relaxation and stress-relief to challenges about food and body that you encounter in everyday life. As a parent, I trust you'll appreciate such an approach.

Guiding Your Children

As parents, you'll be able to address the issues of food, eating, and body image by applying these tips to your whole family. This includes your young children, tweens and teens. As with all endeavors of parenthood, it's your role as parents to determine how best to introduce these concepts to your children. Based on their age, developmental maturity, and temperament, children will vary in their responsiveness to your guidance.

Throughout the full span of childhood, from young child to tween to teen, children will have questions about themselves. Family environment, peer pressure, and cultural influences will all play a role in bringing these questions to the fore. And although not always overtly articulated, parents might hold many of the same questions that children have about themselves. Will she be fat? Is she always going to be this fat? Is he ever going to get taller? Is he not going to lose weight? When will he gain any weight? The tips in this book will help your children search for answers to such questions, and help you as parents guide them in their search.

How to Use this Book

This book is about bringing a voice of balance, trust and joy to your entire life—not just the kitchen or dinning room. Parents and children can explore this book alone or together, as they learn about and have tons of fun with food, eating, and who they are in their bodies. Food is to be embraced, not feared. Our bodies are to be respected, not reviled. Growing up in a world surrounded by positive and healthy attitudes about food and body is the goal.

As you thumb through its pages, I'd like you to keep an open mind and suspend your beliefs about how you think your family might respond to the ideas and tips in this book. When you first try some tips, they might not go over as well or as easily as you would hope. With time and practice, however, I am confident things will click. Give yourself and your family at least three months of practice. Eventually you and your family will discover a new path to thinking about the world of food and body. Allow yourself to be surprised!

Draw on this book as your companion. Bring it to the dinner table or living room to read and enjoy. But also keep it on your nightstand as a reference, for use during those times when topics of food, eating, or body image become thorny for you or your child. Have your children share tips with their friends, and then be prepared to share the knowledge with their parents, as well!

Time to Eat!

As you sit down for the meal that is this book, the table of contents will serve as an excellent menu for selecting those topics you want to consume. The numbered tips are the main course of this book, and I expect you to devour them with passion and gusto! Like a side salad or vegetable, the readings in blue boxes were prepared to supplement the tips, providing extra sustenance on the topic. And for dessert? Well, enjoy Horacio Gatto's wonderful illustrations to bring humor and tasteful grace to compliment your feast.

Bon appétit!

1

Parenting for a Healthy Family Lifestyle

Six Tips About Parenting

1. Never imply with words or actions that your child's weight or body shape is not okay.

2. Never tell your child that she needs to diet.

3. Acknowledge and accept that your own personal views and fears about body and food will influence and sometimes cloud your parental judgment.

4. Your child is not you, and does not have your issues, even if your body types are similar.

5. Issues surrounding food and weight may be a nerve-racking struggle

Room for Improvement

These tips are about refining, enhancing and building on what you already know. Sometimes, just adding a fun activity to the serious matter of feeding our family can make a big difference. There simply is *always* room for improvement as we navigate the pitfalls and challenges of parenthood. Unlearning concepts that were harmful to us as children—that might be harmful to our own children—is part of what this book is all about.

for you, and may influence how you teach your child about such issues.

6. You *can* learn new parenting skills when it comes to food, eating and body image.

Five Tips of Things You Can Do for Your Child

7. Remain positive and supportive of your child, regardless of how much food she ingests and regardless of her body type. She cannot change her body type, and the amount of food she ingests will probably shift in the right direction if you follow these tips.

8. Get out and stay out of your child's plate and stomach. Being on his case will not help the cause.

About the Book's Topics

This book will introduce you to some basic principles about food, the psychology of eating, and body size. Chapter 1 begins with general suggestions for parenting. In chapter 2, you'll learn about how biology influences your child's hunger, with chapter 3 delving more deeply into this topic by exploring how nature and nurture combine to explain why we eat. Chapter 4 is all about food. Chapter 5 explores the good and bad attitudes we have about eating. Chapter 6 turns its attention to the serious topic of bullying, especially as related to weight. And chapter 7 expands on this topic by more closely examining body image. Finally, chapter 8 wraps things up with some general guidelines about eating within the family.

About the Book's Tips

You will learn about the book's topics through a series of tips or suggestions of things you can do for your child, your family, and yourself. Some of these tips may feel outlandish or unattainable. Others may seem unreasonable or irrelevant. Nevertheless, I encourage you to keep reading.

As you progress through the tips, I trust that you'll become more comfortable with the material and it's logic. In the end, the infor- mation will hopefully jell into a complete whole that will help you better understand yourself, your child and your entire family.

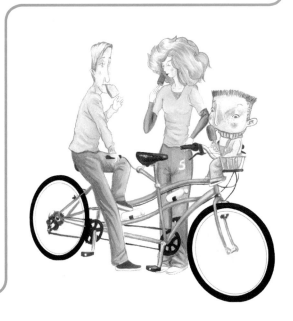

9. Never connect food—any food, not even candy or cake—with fears about weight or body size.

10. Do not make it a big deal when your child eats something un- healthy.

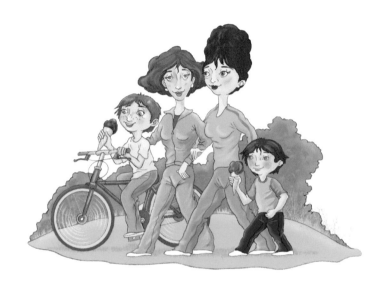

11. Lead by example! Practice healthy, joyful eating—not worrisome, inflammatory eating—making meals a positive, social experience.

2 Self-Regulation

Eight Tips to Help You Discover Self-Regulation

12. Understand and accept that you, the parent, may not have good self-regulation if you grew up in an unhealthy environment regarding food and body image.

13. Trust your child's stomach hunger. After all, you trust her when she is thirsty, right?

14. It's okay to ask your child if she's hungry. *Always* respect her answer.

15. If you cannot control your own eating, it does not mean that you should try to control your child's eating.

16. If you as a parent have a history of eating problems, step back and reflect on how it started. Perhaps at some point your own self-regulation went awry? This

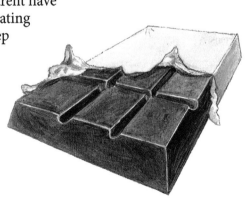

could happen for a number of reasons, and it's worthwhile to explore those social or emotional factors that may have taken control of your eating.

17. Be patient and do not panic if your child overeats or undereats. As your child adjusts to discover his own self-regulation, he may occasionally eat too much or too little until he finds his own equilibrium.

Understanding Self-Regulation

Self-regulation means that your child's biology will control and manage the hunger for food. When most children are left to their own devices—when there is no anxiety, fear or dread attached to eating or its consequences—they are able to start eating when they are hungry and stop eating when they feel they have had enough food. Yes, this is true even when youngsters eat candy or sweets! Children use the feeling in their stomachs to decide if they have had enough to eat. Their eating behavior is governed by a self-regulating system. What this all means is that you, the parent, will need to trust your child's biology.

"No, not my child!" you say?

Before you close this book shaking your head in staunch disagreement, consider the following: Don't you find that you crave exactly what you know you cannot have when faced with an impending diet? When children are threatened with no access to candy until next Halloween, they gorge themselves almost immediately. However, if these same children are made to feel free and secure around sweets, then the chocolate, the frosted cupcakes, and the candy won't have such enticing appeal.

It's All About Trust

When adults hide candy or dish out cake or pizza with the attitude that such foods are dangerous, what they are doing is vesting the rations with power that makes them something not to be missed, something coveted and special. Equally harmful, when we ask children to clean their plates or request that they stop eating because we think they have eaten too much, we are teaching them to mistrust their own bodies. Both requests create children who do not trust their own sense of hunger and satiation.

Consistent with self-regulation, it's important to understand that children have their own unique tastes and food preferences. And they get hungry at certain times but not others. This is normal. This system was not designed to make us mad or angry. It is simply their personal biology, which is something we need to respect to allow health to flourish.

Any time we try to manipulate the hunger–satiation self-regulating system from the *outside*, instead of allowing our children's *inside* biology to manage their food intake as it was designed to do, we risk creating new problems around food and eating.

Accepting Self-Regulation

Following your child's self-regulation isn't easy. Be brave—give it a try! And be patient—give it some time. Eventually, I know you will see results.

18. It takes time to appreciate tomatoes or spinach, especially if they have been pushed nonstop down your throat in the past.

An Exception

One caveat: For some children, self-regulation can be biologically out of balance. For reasons of genetics or disease, they will undereat or overeat when left to their own devices. Although this is not common, it does occasionally happen.

Check with your pediatrician about your child's eating habits and weight if you suspect this to be the case. But be careful to not confuse your own anxiety with a medical matter, or even worse, a medical bias!

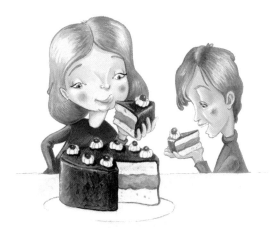

19. Self-regulation is best discovered
    in an environment of love and
    trust.

3

Why Do We Eat?

Five Tips About the Types of Hunger

20. What is *stomach hunger*? This happens when your child feels instinctual or biological hunger. Ask your child: "How do you feel hunger in your stomach?" Swimming butterflies? A grumble? An emptiness? A pain? A void? A lack of energy?

21. What is *eyeball hunger*? This happens when your child sees food and wants to eat, but isn't hungry in the stomach. Ask you child: "Do you ever get hungry

---

Eating as Instinct

Eating is partly an instinctual act. Intuitively we respond to a baby's cry with a desire to feed. It's a primal response.

Our survival is tied to eating. So responding to expressions of hunger with feeding is at the top of the list when we decide to take care of someone.

Intuitively, we think of eating as a behavior determined by biology in support of survival of the species. In other words, virtually all species are born with the capacity to eat. Eating ensures their continued existence.

when we drive past the ice cream store?" Eyeball hunger could be things like seeing candy in a store, passing a pretzel shop at a mall, or seeing a commercial on television for a fast food restaurant. Ask your child to come up with some, as well. Tell your child that what he sees during eyeball hunger is best left to eat during stomach hunger. It will taste better too!

22. What is *emotional hunger*? This happens when your child wants to eat when in a <u>negative mood</u>, like feeling sad, stressed, or upset. Explain to your child that

---

Beyond Instinct

Despite the importance of biology, eating is much more than an instinctual act, and so it may deviate from its original goal for the preservation of life. Beyond instinct, the act of eating has psychological and social underpinnings. These include family dynamics, social pressures or demands, and cultural influences. When eating is no longer about preserving life, we may eat or not eat for other complex reasons that are not connected to the biological hunger signal.

To "look good," perhaps to lose weight before a major family event, we might restrict our eating to an unhealthy degree. To feel more energetic, we might ingest caffeine or other stimulants that go against our normal self-regulation. To increase our muscle mass or tone, we might engage in harmful or excessive exercise that could have unhealthy side effects. We might try to reduce the fat on our bodies and be leaner, even though we are already within a healthy body weight. To disprove or emulate our past or present family dynamics, some of which are not always psychologically healthy, we might change our eating habits.

And the list goes on.

When Psychology Interrupts Biology

When we ascribe a meaning to eating, it may take on a life of its own, and may be linked to psychological or emotional matters that do not necessarily relate to basic survival. Although more common in women than men, many of us have experienced a severing of the biological and psychological purposes of eating. We know about such disconnects when we eat but are not hungry. For instance, most binges and compulsive eating are not related to hunger. They are related to some psychologically pressing issue that does not directly involve hunger or physical survival.

The reverse can occur, as well: When we do not eat, even when hungry, we are responding to matters other than our biology. This might happen if we are trying to diet or have some other reason for limiting our food intake. And in the extreme case, this is what happens during restricted eating, extreme dieting, or anorexia nervosa. Although parents typically wish to avoid these disconnects in a child, they sometimes inadvertently and paradoxically facilitate them when manipulating a child's food intake.

certain feelings such as being upset or bored could sometimes make her want to eat, even when not hungry in the stomach. Ask your child: "Do you ever want to eat when you are not hungry? Or do you ever get hungry when you are in a certain mood?" Bad mood? Good mood? Sad mood? Happy mood? Emotional hunger could follow feelings of doubt, fear, boredom, disgust, anger, or nervousness. Ask your child to come up with some, as well. Try to present your child with outlets for her feelings other than eating, like playing ball, listening to music, or talking.

23. Teach your child to be a *hunger detective.* Have her learn to pay attention to what she is feeling when she gets hungry. Tell her she should have a conversation with her stomach! Practice finding *eyeball clues* for eyeball hunger, and *emotional cues* for emotional hunger. Make it into a fun game!

24. Ask your daughter whether she would like to choose an activity other than eating when she feels eye hunger or emotional hunger. What could it be? Be creative and help her out. But do not pressure her if she still decides to eat.

Four Tips About Your Child's Relationship with Food

25. Make a list of the foods your son wants you to buy. Now go to the store and purchase them. Okay, go ahead and cringe a little. Now that you're done cringing, *purchase them!* Your son will begin to trust his stomach and you. And yes, you will be asked to buy candy, chips, cakes, double stuffed pizza, and all sorts of snack food. You will be tested mightily on whether you really let him buy such food. And you will also be tested on whether you really let him eat such food once you bring it home. Be patient and trust his hunger.

26. Allow your daughter to determine the amount of food that goes on her plate.

27. Do not judge, argue about, or change the amount of food in your child's hands.

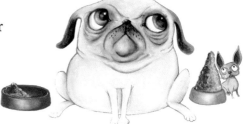

Your New Approach to Eating

When working to create a healthy family food environment, children and parents need to learn an approach that will help each member of the family be happier when it comes to eating. It's an approach based on trust of everyone's stomach and sense of hunger. In this way of relating, each family member is in charge of his or her own stomach.

How does this new approach work? Well, it's fairly simple. This is the fundamental rule: *You eat when you are hungry.* Things taste better when you experience stomach hunger.

From time to time, all of us will eat when not hungry. This is normal. But if we eat to excess on a daily basis, or almost always restrict our eating to an extreme, then this is not healthy eating. If this occurs for you or your child, it's important for you both to do some detective work.

28. Always ask your son whether he is hungry when he says he wants to eat. *Trust* the answer. It is for *him* to say, not you. Avoid assessing hunger in a police-like manner. Rather, build trust between the two of you, to discover your child's self-regulation. This cannot be stressed enough: Following this tip will allow your child to grow up to be a healthy eater. A healthy eater is a person who can follow his stomach hunger regarding *when* he wants to eat, *what* he wants to eat, and *how much* he wants to eat, from the inside out.

This Is Detective Work

As detectives, you and your child will try to uncover and explore those feelings that may lurk under the desire to eat when not hungry, or to avoid eating when hungry. Sometimes the reasons are simple and normal: That chocolate truffle looks *so* scrumptious that you just *have* to have it! You eat one and are done.

But sometimes the reasons are more complex and hidden. For example, if you grew up in a very unhealthy family environment, you might not understand the many factors that could influence your hunger. The tips in this section will help you and your child to become your own detectives, to understand the underlying psychological causes of hunger.

Four Tips About Satiation

29. Satiation is a distinct, comfortable feeling in the stomach. It says: "That hit the spot, and I do not want any more food." This is not necessarily the same thing as "feeling full."

Satiation

Closely related to the perception of hunger is the feeling of *satiation*, which is the reduction and ultimate disappearance of hunger. Satiation is the terminus of self-regulation. It is the natural and automatic switch that signals the body to stop eating.

However, modern accessibility to food, the proliferation of processed and junk foods, and the sociocultural imperative to diet and restrict food intake can distort our satiation, throwing off our self-regulation. "Do not eat too much!" is the commandment that has perverted this mechanism.

Unfortunately, some cannot discern when they are satiated and need to stop eating. Some start eating when they are not physically hungry. Others keep eating when they are very full. Some continue eating past their feelings of fullness. Others reach for food when they are stressed. An unhealthy dynamic gets established between the physical and emotional needs of a person. And we teach our children to do the same.

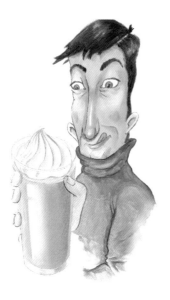

30. Most children are excellent at knowing when they've had enough to eat.

31. Do not tamper with your child's innate healthy satiation mechanism. Avoid a steadfast rule of requiring a child to empty his plate. Likewise, avoid telling your child to stop eating before feeling satiated.

32. Trust your child's natural satiation point. Don't try to change it. Rather, help your child understand what it feels like. Your children can understand their natural satiation point only if they know that they'll be able to eat what they like, on their own terms. If they don't have a handle on their natural satiation point, they will almost surely gorge when you aren't around.

Getting Back In Touch

A healthy lifestyle and healthy eating mandates that we get back in touch with both our hunger and our satiation. They represent the body's natural signals of when to start and stop eating.

Teach your children to pay attention to how it feels when they are satisfied, and that the feeling is a signal to stop eating.

4

All About Food

Eight Tips About Nutritious Foods & Snacks

33. Nutritious foods, sometimes called wholesome foods, help us accomplish desirable things for our bodies by keeping us strong and healthy. Explain this to your youngster.

34. Nutritious foods do *not* always taste bad—that's a myth. They can be quite scrumptious! Work with your children to find out which nutritious foods appeal to them. Get them involved in the selection and make it fun!

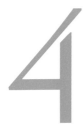

35. Eating nutritious foods should quench most of one's stomach hunger.

36. A snack is food to hold you over until the next meal. Although a snack can be any size, you can teach your child that the next meal will taste better if she is hungry in her stomach. Don't set any ironclad rule about its size or kind. Your child's stomach is the boss, not you. Her stomach will ultimately select the correct amount and variety, once she doesn't have to battle you for a piece of chocolate.

37. Teach your child that she will enjoy dinner more if she limits here snacks and is moderately hungry when the next meal arrives. Children may be ravenous when they return from school, and this is especially true for tweens and teens. It doesn't respect their biology to force them to wait until dinner without providing a snack. Although it is true that your child will be

Defining Food

What is food? What is a snack? These days, edibles come in many unrecognizable packages with many unrecognizable ingredients and names. Sometimes, those edibles we purchase are nutritious foods. More often than not, the best food is what we prepare at home with ingredients we know to be fresh, natural, and chemical-free, making it tasty and generally nutritious.

Sometimes edible matter has limited nutritional value. If something is filled with chemicals and preservatives, I wouldn't even call it food! Rather it's a laboratory-perfected, mass-produced concoction designed to fool our palate into thinking it's good for us when it's actually bad for our bodies. Of course it is good for something, namely a sector of the economy that competes for your attention over fresh fruits and vegetables. Such concoctions, if consumed to excess, can deceive our biology and throw off our self-regulation. This is not a good thing.

> ## *Managing "Junk Food"*
>
> Despite the danger of laboratory-produced edibles (sometimes called "junk food," though I hate the term), it's *not* a good idea to impose an outright ban on such products. Do that, and our children will learn that they're enticing forbidden foods to sneak into their mouths.
>
> It's better to define such edibles as being once-in-a-while treats, to be occasionally consumed within the normal course of life. It's a good idea to help our children understand that although some foods might taste *really good*, eating too much of them can be *really bad* for their health. Ultimately it is best to allow your children to learn by making their own choices.

hungrier and probably enjoy dinner more if pre-dinner snacks are limited, this is for her to discover in a relaxed, pressure-free environment.

38. Help your child differentiate between normal hunger and starvation. How? By quantifying their stomach hunger on a scale from one to ten.

39. Plan and tailor snacks to provide variety and appeal to the tastes of your children.

40. Work with your son to come up with tasty wholesome snacks. Make a list and go shopping together. Who will be the bravest to try something new? Salt-dried peas? Organic gum? Take some fun playful risks, and maybe you'll find a new tasty food!

Five Tips About the Sweet Tooth

41. There is no crime in having a sweet tooth. It's not a bad thing.

Food Freedom

As our children age into their tween and teen years, you will no doubt find that they will lament that they don't have as much freedom and control as they would like. And here is one area where you may consider empowering your tween or teen with control over food.

They are generally very good at figuring out how much food is too much or too little. Your job is to curb your own anxiety and allow them to discover their own self-regulatory equilibrium. Getting attuned to one's body won't happen overnight. Be patient, and it will eventually come to pass.

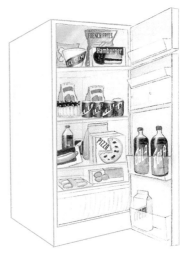

42. Teach your child that she always has choices when it comes to food and eating. She can save a hunger space for sweets (like candy) and a hunger space for nutritious food (like fruit). Having choices, instead of directives, will allow her to better connect with her stomach hunger and eat accordingly.

43. As a parent, eat sweets and enjoy them. And enjoy your vegetables, too. Through example, teach your

child that it can be fun to eat all kinds of foods without feeling guilty or making a big deal out of it.

44. Make having sweets a fun part of life!

45. Avoid an absolutist approach by banning certain foods. It will only make your child want them more.

Five Tips for Healthy Eating

46. Bring your child with you to the grocery store to help you buy food. Go together and make it a fun expedition to find foods that both of you like. Experiment with healthy versus unhealthy, yummy versus yucky, organic versus processed. Teach your child that you trust him and his inner decision-making system regarding food. Who knows? He may surprise you by choosing edamame!

47. You promote healthy eating when your child is not afraid that you might go ballistic over what he ate.

The Sweet Tooth

Laboratory-produced edibles are high in calories, low in nutrients, and filled with chemicals, colorants or preservatives. Because these foods are designed and manufactured to be tasty to the human palate and often contain sugars, they are especially appealing to children. Hence we say kids have a sweet tooth. But this makes children especially vulnerable to crave nutritionally limited foods.

However, there is a way to appease the desire for sweets. As your child learns to eat by respecting stomach hunger, the desire for sweets will wane. Her stomach will eventually recognize the need for nutritional proteins and vegetables.

Healthy Eating

It is beyond the scope of this book to provide specific advice about what foods to buy or eat. For such advice, it's best to consult a nutritionist or doctor. However there are some basic principles to follow when selecting foods. Ultimately, you will make the final decision of what goes into your mouth, and you are the most significant role model for what your children put into their mouths.

We all know that fruits and vegetables are healthy and a good choice for you and your family. If you regularly include such natural foods in your diet, you are already on the correct pathway to healthy eating.

Healthy eating also means the following: You consume a variety of foods without fear, anxiety, obligation, or coercion. The hallmark of healthy eating in family life is flexibility, and not managing or controlling what lies in each other's plates. The hallmark of healthy relating in family life is not being judgmental about each other's physical appearance.

48. Accept that your child can handle looking at sweets without gorging on them (unless maybe, if it's Halloween, and it means feasting with friends).

49. Do *not* make a big deal about your child's appropriately restrictive taste. Some children have seemingly restrictive eating habits by avoiding variety. This is perfectly natural and due to taste, not fear or dieting.

50. Understand that children expand their food horizons when they reach 9 or 10 years of age, and you do not need to interfere with such development.

5 Bad Attitudes

Five Tips to Avoid Negative Attitudes

51. Try to avoid holding this bad attitude: "I do not buy any sweets or junk food because my child cannot control her eating of such food." By holding such a view, you're not allowing your child's natural self-regulation to guide her eating. You're also sending a message of distrust that your child is likely to detect. Dispense with this attitude and try to become more relaxed with your child's food choices.

52. Avoid shaming by holding this bad attitude: "I weigh my child often so she knows she has to keep an eye on herself." Weigh-ins only promote a fear of judgment—the feeling that one is not okay with how one is—and hang-ups about weight!

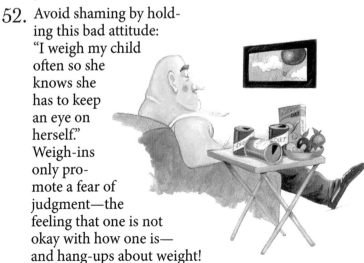

Weigh-ins also create false hope ("Hooray, I lost a pound!") or foster dejection ("Shucks, I'm getting fat again."). Basically, you do not want your child's happiness to be tied to the number in a scale. Self-esteem must not depend on weight!

53. Do not do the following: "I tell my child that he has to exercise to keep in shape." Although exercise is healthy, the requirement to "keep in shape" puts unnecessary pressure on a child, and exercise should not be associated with pressure or mandates. Exercise without labeling it. Incorporate it in your daily routine without focusing on an ulterior motive (like losing weight). Walk the dog or park the farther away from the store. Try to find an activity your child actually likes, even if it is not

What Is an Attitude?

We tell our children not to have a "bad attitude," when they talk back to us disrespectfully, or when they roll their eyes. We try to reinforce "good attitudes" of industriousness, respect, and kindness. Fundamentally, an attitude is a strongly held belief or thought about some issue.

Children of all ages and adults can portray attitudes through what they say (verbally) or how they act (nonverbally). A boy can bully the fat kid by shoving him. A girl can engage in relational bullying by insinuating that someone is "fat," or by gossiping about someone's weight. But words are not always necessary: An aversion of the eyes or a disparaging look can suffice to portray a certain attitude.

> ### *Attitudes About Food, Eating, & Body Image*
>
> Most of us have strongly held attitudes about food, eating, and body image. Often we learn such beliefs as children. And society is not very helpful with challenging those strongly held attitudes: "Beautiful and thin" are united just like "fat and ugly" always seem to go together. Regrettably, many such attitudes are irrational and the behaviors that follow can be destructive to others. Negative parental attitudes about food, eating, or body image can get in the way of healthy family relations. Negative parental attitudes about body size are harmful to those we love.

gender "appropriate." So what if he likes to dance and she likes karate?

54. Steer clear of embarrassing your child, tween or teen: "One look from me and she immediately knows she should not be eating that." By having such an attitude, you're destructively controlling your child's eating, making her feel like she's under the watchful eye of a food dictator. You might also make her feel like she's eating too much (even though she's not) or make her feel that she's fat (even though she's not). And holding such attitudes might even lower her self-esteem.

55. Avoid criticizing yourself by saying, "I feel guilty—I ate *so* much." Or, "Gee, I look *so* fat! Or, "I should *so* go on a diet." Children, tweens and teens are like sponges that soak up everything you say and often turn your attitudes into their own.

Seven Tips to Foster Positive Attitudes

56. Eating should happen from the inside out. This means that feelings of hunger and satiation should come from the *inside*, from your child's awareness of his biology as directed by natural self-regulation, instead of from *outside* influences following the social pressure of parents or peers.

57. Make an effort to enjoy food together. Involve your children in cooking for fun. Do you remember roasting s'mores over a campfire? Those were fun to prepare and healthy to consume because the social environment was fun and healthy.

58. Children, teens, and tweens love to eat the food that *they* prepare. Let them do it!

59. Do not become a kitchen slave. Simplify your life in the kitchen. Get a Crockpot. Use a microwave. Select wholesome menus that require minimal effort. Make it easy and fun to cook, not a chore.

60. Repeat after me: "I am not what I cook." Do not allow your self-esteem to be affected by how your food is received by your family. Remember that you are wonderful for many reasons! So if someone doesn't like what you cooked, it is not a personal rejection.

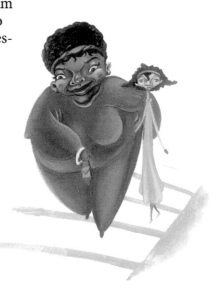

61. Enjoy what you eat! If you like ice cream or cookies, don't be bashful about telling your family. Likewise, if you enjoy eating your spinach salad, be sure to let them know this, as well.

62. Do not talk about dieting with your children. Dieting is all about restricting or limiting your food intake, and this *not* an approach to food you want to promote.

What Is a Diet Mentality?

If you manipulate your food intake because of an underlying fear of gaining weight, you have what is called a *diet mentality*. It is one example of a negative attitude about food and eating that is worth avoiding.

Four Tips to Avoid a Diet Mentality

63. If you believe that you need to be strict about what your child eats, because you believe that being strict is important for his health, it's a form of diet mentality. In fact, you may be putting your child's health at risk by creating a psychological state of worry around food.

64. Question those beliefs you hold that tell you that eating in a certain, prescribed manner is always the right thing to do. By being rigid and inflexible about your child's eating styles, or by strictly enforcing how to eat or how much to eat, you are defining a very narrow range of permissible eating behavior for your child. Ultimately, you are interfering with self-regulation.

65. Do not enforce strict food portions. By severely limiting your family's portions, you undermine natural

self-regulation and rob your child from getting to know her own body and the clues it gives her.

66. Never plan snacks according to how your child will "burn them off." Here you may be taking unnecessarily obsessive control over your child's metabolism. If you allow your child to have the freedom to move, you will find out that when the human body is unhindered by social restriction, it is a fantastic machine that can work its magic. It's better to curtail sedentary time (like using the computer or watching television) to provide an opportunity for your child to engage in natural movement.

6

All About Bullying

Six Tips About People Who Bully

67. Make it clear to your child that friends who taunt him about food, weight or body shape may not realize that their "joking" is making him feel bad.

68. Inform your child that no one is entitled to mistreat her, even if they are going though a hard time themselves. There are no justifications or excuses for bullying.

69. Although bullying is intentional, some kids don't have a good sense of *how* harmful bullying can be to others. This is partly why they keep doing it. Explain this to your child, and let her know this is true for some kids who bully.

70. Let your child know that it's unfortunate that some kids think they can get away with hurting other people's feelings. And this is partly why they keep doing it. Encourage your child to find new friends. Discourage him from remaining friends with people who regularly put him or others down.

71. Teach your child that when someone bullies another, they are trying to exercise power over that person. This is partly why they keep doing it. By getting in-

What Is Bullying?

The tips in this chapter were written for you as a parent to help your child, tween, and teen when they encounter offensive and demeaning behavior from a peer. This is commonly known as bullying, and can take many forms including verbal, nonverbal, and physical variants. Bullying can be delivered many ways, including in person, on paper, as graffiti on bathroom walls, on a Web site, over the telephone, and via text message. Bullying is done intentionally to inflict harm on another person.

Kids can be bullied for all sorts of reasons, and some of the most common are related to their body size or shape. What they eat, how they eat, and with whom they eat can also be targets for the bully. So it's important to be knowledgeable about your child's life away from home, and how peer interactions in your child's life can sometimes go awry.

volved with new people and new activities, your child will take that power away.

72. Cultivate empathy in your home. Making fun of others is a bad habit and harmful to others. *Don't do it.*

Six Tips On How to Confront Those Who Bully

73. Help your child be strong and assertive. Help her be clear about what words make her feel bad and what behaviors she wants the bully to stop doing. Practice with her so she can be brief and sound secure when talking to the bully.

Teasing versus Bullying

It is different to be teased than to be bullied. Teasing is usually done for humor among friends, and the person doing the teasing along with the person being teased are usually good friends, and they laugh *with* each other. Usually no one gets offended or feels bad once the teasing is over.

But bullying is altogether something else! Teasing is about having *constructive fun* with someone. Bullying is about having *destructive power* over someone.

Bullying is a very serious matter. With bullying, people are laughing *at* you instead of with you. There is nothing funny about bullying. In fact, the person being bullied feels *horrible*! Bullying can easily escalate to harmful actions.

74. Tell your child that if a friend doesn't stop making fun of her after several requests to stop, she must find a new friend.

75. If your child feels taunted or ridiculed about her weight, she needs to get the help of a trusted adult.

76. Remind your child that when someone is truly mean to her, she has the right to tell a trusted adult about what is happening.

77. There is a big difference between "telling" and being a "tattletale." The purpose of being a *tattletale* is to get *others* in trouble. The purpose of *telling* is to seek help for *yourself*.

78. Talk to your children about participating in community work that benefits others and instills values to

---

What Can Kids Do?

If your child is being bullied, her safety may be at stake. In fact, if you feel that someone is bullying her, tell her to follow these steps:

1. Get yourself away from the people who are bullying you. Your physical safety comes first.
2. Call a trusted adult for guidance, and let them know everything that happened. They are here to help you.
3. Contact your school guidance office for help.
4. Call a close friend for support.
5. If you cannot get away or are still in immediate danger, call the police.

Almost all schools have policies against bullying. Indeed, many schools have an anti-bullying movement with which your child can get involved. Remind your child that she is not alone!

promote supportive social acceptance and productive friendships. Suggest that they help others help themselves by starting a new club, such as Kids Against Bullying.

Five Tips On What to Do When Bullied

79. When your child feels bad about himself, have him sit down in a quiet room and make a list of five qualities that he likes about his own personality. Then ask him to make a list of five physical features that he likes in himself. Encourage him: "You can do it!" You can even review your child's list, providing positive feedback and recognition of these positive characteristics.

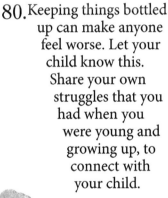

80. Keeping things bottled up can make anyone feel worse. Let your child know this. Share your own struggles that you had when you were young and growing up, to connect with your child.

81. Remind your child that he has the *power* to do something about his situation, and that this is only a temporary phase in his life. Ask him to follow the steps in the "What Can Kids Do?" box.

82. Help your child understand that he needn't feel trapped by unfriendly people. As a parent, let him know that he has choices, can take action against bullying, and can make new friends.

Stay Aware of Bullying

Being bullied hurts and is embarrassing, so your child may not
tell you about it right away. Look for
behaviors such as low grades, isola-
tion, sadness, and irritability. If your
child is starving after school, bullies may
be taking his lunch away. If you notice
that your child starts avoiding many
social activities, he may be trying to evade
bullies. Watch especially for a significant
change in your child's behavior.

One of the best ways to catch bullying
early is to keep an open line of communication
with your child, discussing what goes on in his
life when away from home. As a parent, never
normalize or diminish a situation when your child
says he is being bullied. A teacher, school counsel-
or, or another parent may be best equipped to talk
with you about your own unique situation.

83. In the face of adversity, help your child
discover the good things about himself.
This will strengthen his self-esteem and
make him better able to address the
bullying.

If Your Child Is Being Bullied

If you learn of a specific episode of bullying, talk to your child when he is calm and can convey clear information about what happened. Give him your strong support and remind him that this is a temporary situation. Let him know that there is always a way out, which will provide him with hope that things will change for the better.

As a parent, you also need support, so speak with a close friend who is also a parent to get guidance and perspective. You also will need to speak with a school official to find out what happened and to relate your child's version of the events to the school. The school should be there to help you. When you tell the school what happened to your child, provide clear examples. Be a positive agent of change for your child and the school. It's usually not helpful to act in an adversarial manner. Work with school officials to ensure the bullying stops.

7

Body Image

Nine Tips About Body Image

84. The negative picture we have of ourselves is seldom related to how we look or what we eat.

85. Children grow to unduly care about body image if they see us obsessed with it.

86. See the beauty in your child, even if he is not stereotypically beautiful.

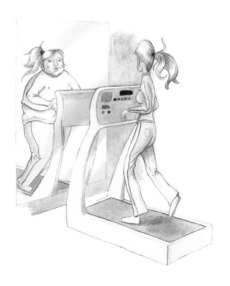

What Is Body Image?

Body image is the picture that we hold inside our mind about how our own body looks. It is what we know about ourselves, even before we look in the mirror. Body image is related to self-esteem, which is how we feel about ourselves as an overall person.

Because of the relationship between body image and self-esteem, sometimes our minds do not hold an accurate image of how we look physically. Many parents know this phenomenon well: They felt fat at some point in their lives. But when they look at pictures from that era, they see (to great surprise!) that they were actually quite thin.

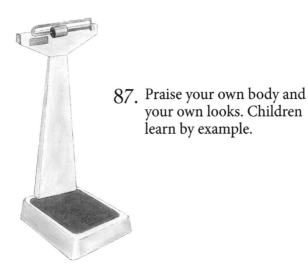

87. Praise your own body and
    your own looks. Children
    learn by example.

88. If you help your child feel funny, smart,
    witty, loving, friendly, strong, secure
    and loved, then how their body looks
    will not become their primary concern.

89. Parental eyes that *see* beauty make your
    child *feel* beautiful.

Where Does Body Image Come From?

Body image is not something that children are born with. It is acquired as they grow up and it is closely related to how they feel about themselves as a whole. Because of this, it is important that we give our children the best possible start. It is crucial that we make them feel okay and comfortable about their own bodies, no matter what size they might be.

Furthermore, it takes a good number of years for children to actually *care* about how they look. This works to parents' advantage since it gives mothers and fathers time to foster security, strength, and healthy self-esteem in their children before body self-perceptions begin to take shape.

90. Tell your child about her outer beauty. Make your child aware of those unique physical characteristics of her body that are beautiful. Despite all we often hear about the value of inner beauty, we all also possess outer beauty. Don't be modest!

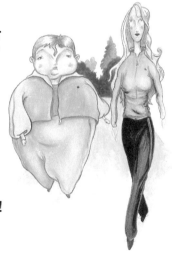

91. Find role models for your child that look like him.

92. Discover beauty in difference.

The Ugly Phantom

For many parents, their own body image is an *ugly phantom*—a leftover presence of youth from which they want to spare their child. For others, peace around the topic of their own body image has been won after hard work. Unfortunately, wanting to spare our child our own body image misfortune is what, paradoxically, may cause the most trouble!

It is not in our child's best interest to superimpose our own body image experience onto theirs, because a child's body image is in flux and under continuous development. Furthermore, they are bound to have a *different* body image because they experience *different* environments, have *different* friends, and are reared by *different* parents than us.

8 Family Life & Eating

Seven Tips for Healthy Family Eating

93. Eat together, not alone.

94. Engage in conversations at mealtime, and involve the whole family including the children. Avoid heavy topics or serious issues while dining, which are best handled at separate times.

95. Eliminate anything that can distract from eating and conversation, such as televisions or other electronic devices.

96. Don't enforce rigid eating schedules or unexamined customs. A small healthy snack in the afternoon can make the difference between a peaceful meal and World War III at dinnertime.

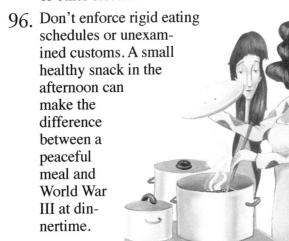

The Complexity of Eating

Living life as a family is not always easy. There are busy schedules that don't always jive. There are competing preferences about what family members like to do for fun. And there are the normal and natural conflicts members have with each other as they navigate their individual lives. But one activity that everyone *must* engage in is eating.

Eating within the family is not as easy as it would first seem. Eating can be complicated because it is an instinctual, an individual, and a social act. Why would an act as primitive as eating be fraught with so many complexities?

97. Once in a while, change the time of day! Cook breakfast for dinner.

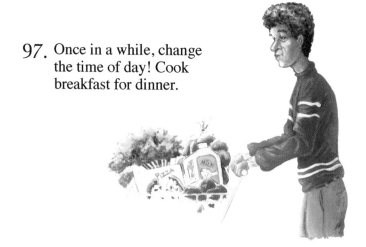

Early Eating Relationships

Eating is the first act we do in the context of a relationship. With our eating, we internalize complex patterns of relating to each other. For example, an infant's eating happens within the context of a relationship between a baby and caregiver. It always has been that way because babies need someone to feed them. And many people can feed babies: mother, father, relatives, and even wet nurses or other caregivers. So our earliest relationships in life involve eating.

Those who feed us and those who raise us shape who we are and how we behave. This is part of what defines our developing personality. An anxious father, for instance, might hold the bottle in a certain manner, maybe tentatively, as if scared. A hurried one might communicate time pressure by rushing a feeding. A depressed mother might often look away, though one who is attuned would cast appropriate and loving glances at the baby. A laid back caregiver in turn, might convey her feeling of relaxation to the infant. Our early eating relationships are so important that even mythology informs us about a caring wolf that nursed the brothers Romulus and Remus, who later gave birth to ancient Rome.

Ingesting More than Food

A developing child will ingest more than just food when eating. A certain atmosphere, a certain environment, a certain mood, and a certain way of relating are all part of the eating process. The child will learn that eating comes with a specific set of sensations, passions and feelings. So in the context of our relationships, we connect emotions to eating. Growing up, we might learn that eating alone is sad. Or perhaps it is full of pressure and rushing. Or we might learn that we can only be happy while eating alone. We develop strong emotions around eating. We might learn to be ashamed of how much or how little we eat.

What happens in these cases is that we no longer eat by self-regulation, the body's natural rhythm of hunger and satiation (see chapter 1). Rather, we eat according to how we think others might *judge* our eating. So when it comes time for us to sit down at the family table, it's important to recognize that no one arrives with a truly empty plate! Every person at the table has a unique relationship with food, and that relationship will be different from that of every other person. These differences have the potential to disrupt an otherwise harmonious family meal.

Eating Within a Family

If you now eat separately as a family, I suggest you begin to have *at least* one meal together, around a single table. Ensure that there are no other distractions, such as television, smart phones, laptops, electronic tablets, books, or newspapers, unless they enhance the existing conversation at the table. And talk. Yes, talk, converse, communicate, relate. Your goal is to develop and enhance your family relationships as you eat.

For food, provide basic staples because children will not always feel as adventurous as adults. It's okay if your child wants to eat the same thing for a whole week. The acceptance of a variety of foods will happen faster if you do not mandate new foods. Of course, continue to provide a choice of new, unique, and adventurous foods. This way your child will see other foods being served at the home. Occasionally encourage your child to try something new, without pressure.

98. Once in a while, eat backwards! Start with dessert and end with the appetizer.

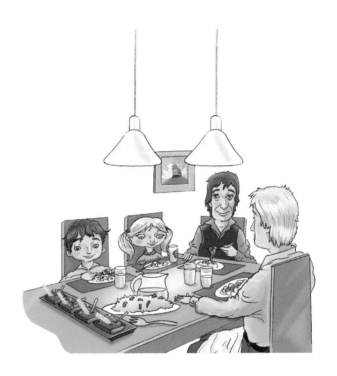

99. Finally, in essence, make the family eating experience fun and enjoyable!

Approaching Harmony

Fortunately we are not solely determined by our early eating relationships. Mercifully, our eating experiences are part of a complex developmental process that can be changed at many different points in time. And these changes can be made well into adulthood, through our continued experiences and relationships. It is this potential for change that gives us hope.

A healthy family environment will transform this hope into reality. Family is the vehicle where we can change the negative emotions that may exist around the eating experience. Through what we do in a family, we develop a more harmonious eating environment for our children, our family, our friends, and ultimately all whom we encounter in life.

CPSIA information can be obtained
at www.ICGtesting.com
Printed in the USA
BVIC00n0016181114
374700BV00001B/1